UNMASKING HYPERTENSION: THE TRUTH ABOUT HIGH BLOOD PRESSURE AND PROVEN SOLUTIONS FOR PREVENTION

Introduction:

- The importance of understanding high blood pressure

Understanding high blood pressure is of paramount importance for several reasons. Here is a detailed explanation of why it is crucial to have a comprehensive understanding of this condition:

High blood pressure, also known as hypertension, is a prevalent health concern globally. According to the World Health Organization (WHO), hypertension affects approximately 1.13 billion people worldwide. It is a major risk factor for cardiovascular diseases, including heart attacks, strokes, and heart failure. Understanding high blood pressure helps individuals recognize its significance and take appropriate measures to prevent or manage it.

One of the primary reasons for understanding high blood pressure is its silent nature. It often does not exhibit noticeable symptoms in its early stages, leading to the term "silent killer." Many people may have hypertension without even realizing it. By understanding high blood pressure, individuals can appreciate the need for regular blood pressure monitoring and early detection to prevent complications.

Hypertension poses various health risks. It can damage blood vessels, leading to atherosclerosis, which is the narrowing of the arteries. This increases the risk of heart disease and stroke. High blood pressure also strains the heart, causing it to work harder and potentially leading to heart failure. Understanding these risks motivates individuals to adopt preventive measures, make lifestyle changes, and seek appropriate medical care.

Understanding the risk factors associated with high blood pressure is essential for prevention and management. While some risk factors, such as age, family history, and genetics, cannot be modified, lifestyle factors significantly contribute to the development of hypertension. Poor diet, physical inactivity, smoking, excessive alcohol consumption, and obesity are some of the modifiable risk factors. By understanding these risk factors, individuals can make informed choices and reduce their chances of developing high blood pressure.

Another reason for understanding high blood pressure is empowerment and self-care. By being aware of the condition, individuals can actively participate in their healthcare, make informed decisions, and take necessary steps to prevent or manage hypertension. This includes adopting a healthy lifestyle, monitoring blood pressure regularly, and complying with medical treatment, if required.

High blood pressure does not only affect cardiovascular health but also impacts overall well-being. It can contribute to kidney damage, vision problems, cognitive decline, and sexual dysfunction. Understanding the far-reaching consequences of hypertension motivates individuals to prioritize their health and make choices that support overall well-being.

Prevention is key when it comes to high blood pressure. Understanding the condition helps individuals recognize the importance of preventive measures. Maintaining a healthy weight, eating a balanced diet, engaging in regular physical activity, managing stress, limiting sodium intake, and avoiding smoking and excessive alcohol consumption are some of the preventive strategies. By taking proactive steps, individuals can reduce their risk of developing hypertension and its associated complications.

In summary, understanding high blood pressure is vital due to its prevalence, silent nature, health risks, genetic predisposition, empowerment, impact on overall health, and the importance of prevention. By gaining knowledge about hypertension, individuals can make informed decisions, seek appropriate medical care, and take proactive measures to prevent or manage this condition effectively. It is essential to spread awareness about the significance of understanding high blood pressure to promote healthier lives and reduce the burden of cardiovascular diseases.

- Explaining the prevalence and impact of hypertension in modern society

Hypertension, commonly known as high blood pressure, is a prevalent and impactful health condition in modern society. Understanding its prevalence and impact is crucial for addressing this global health concern effectively. Here is a detailed explanation of the prevalence and impact of hypertension:

Prevalence:
Hypertension is a widespread health issue affecting a significant portion of the global population. According to the World Health Organization (WHO), approximately 1.13 billion people worldwide have hypertension. This accounts for about 1 in 4 adults. The prevalence of hypertension increases with age, and it is more common in low and middle-income countries. The rising prevalence of hypertension is attributed to various factors, including sedentary lifestyles, unhealthy diets, obesity, and an aging population.

Impact on Cardiovascular Health:
Hypertension is a major risk factor for cardiovascular diseases, including heart attacks, strokes, and heart failure. Elevated blood pressure levels can damage blood vessels, leading to atherosclerosis,

which is the buildup of plaque in the arteries. This restricts blood flow and increases the risk of heart disease. Additionally, hypertension strains the heart, making it work harder to pump blood, which can eventually lead to heart failure. The impact of hypertension on cardiovascular health is significant, making it a leading cause of morbidity and mortality worldwide.

Impact on Kidney Health:
Hypertension can have detrimental effects on kidney health. Prolonged high blood pressure can damage the blood vessels in the kidneys, impairing their ability to filter waste and excess fluid from the body. This can lead to chronic kidney disease and, in severe cases, kidney failure. Hypertension-related kidney disease is a significant cause of end-stage renal disease, requiring dialysis or kidney transplantation for survival. Managing blood pressure is essential to preserve kidney function and prevent the progression of kidney disease.

Impact on Brain Health:
Untreated or poorly controlled hypertension increases the risk of cerebrovascular diseases, such as strokes and vascular dementia. High blood pressure can cause damage to the blood vessels in the brain, leading to ischemic strokes (caused by blood clots) or hemorrhagic strokes (caused by bleeding in the brain). Strokes can result in long-term disability, cognitive impairment, and even death. Hypertension is also associated with an increased risk of vascular dementia, a condition characterized by a decline in cognitive abilities due to reduced blood flow and damage to the brain.

Impact on Overall Health:
Hypertension not only affects specific organs but also has a broader impact on overall health. It is associated with an increased risk of other health conditions, including diabetes, metabolic syndrome, sleep apnea, and certain types of cancer. Hypertension can also exacerbate existing health conditions, making management more challenging. Moreover, it can reduce the quality of life, leading to physical limitations, psychological distress, and decreased productivity.

Economic and Social Impact:
The impact of hypertension extends beyond individual health. It places a significant economic burden on healthcare systems and society as a whole. The costs associated with the diagnosis, treatment, and management of hypertension, as well as its complications, are substantial. Furthermore, hypertension-related hospitalizations, disability, and premature deaths result in productivity losses and reduced quality of life for individuals and their families. Addressing hypertension on a societal level is essential to mitigate these economic and social impacts.

In summary, hypertension is a prevalent and impactful health condition in modern society. Its high prevalence, particularly in low and middle-income countries, coupled with its profound impact on cardiovascular health, kidney health, brain health, and overall well-being, makes it a significant global health concern. Understanding the prevalence and impact of hypertension is crucial for implementing effective prevention, early detection, and management strategies to reduce the burden of this condition and improve the health outcomes of individuals and communities.

Chapter 1: Understanding High Blood Pressure

- Defining high blood pressure and its causes

High blood pressure, also known as hypertension, is a medical condition characterized by elevated blood pressure levels in the arteries. Blood pressure is the force exerted by the blood against the walls of the blood vessels as the heart pumps it throughout the body. It is measured using two values: systolic pressure (the force when the heart beats) and diastolic pressure (the force when the heart is at rest between beats). Normal blood pressure is typically around 120/80 mmHg (millimeters of mercury) or lower.

High blood pressure is a significant health concern due to its prevalence and the impact it has on cardiovascular health, kidney health, brain health, and overall well-being. Understanding the causes of high blood pressure is crucial for effective prevention, early detection, and management strategies.

There are two types of high blood pressure: primary (essential) hypertension and secondary hypertension.

1. Primary (Essential) Hypertension:
Primary hypertension is the most common type, accounting for about 90-95% of cases. The exact cause of primary hypertension is often unknown, but it is believed to be a result of a combination of genetic and environmental factors. Risk factors associated with primary hypertension include:

Age: The risk of developing hypertension increases with age. As people get older, the blood vessels become less elastic, making it harder for blood to flow through them.

Family history: Having a family history of hypertension increases the likelihood of developing the condition. Genetic factors can contribute to an individual's susceptibility to high blood pressure.

Lifestyle factors: Unhealthy lifestyle choices can contribute to the development of hypertension. These include a high-sodium diet, lack of physical activity, excessive alcohol consumption, and tobacco use. A diet high in sodium can cause the body to retain fluid, increasing blood volume and, subsequently, blood pressure. Physical inactivity can lead to weight gain and increased strain on the heart, while excessive alcohol consumption and tobacco use can damage blood vessels and raise blood pressure.

Obesity: Being overweight or obese puts extra strain on the heart and blood vessels, increasing the risk of hypertension. Adipose tissue produces various hormones and inflammatory substances that can interfere with blood pressure regulation.

Insulin resistance and metabolic syndrome: Insulin resistance, a condition in which the body's cells do not respond properly to insulin, and metabolic syndrome, a cluster of conditions that include high blood pressure, high blood sugar, abnormal cholesterol levels, and excess abdominal fat, are closely associated with the development of hypertension.

2. Secondary Hypertension:
Secondary hypertension is caused by an underlying medical condition or certain medications. It accounts for about 5-10% of hypertension cases. Some common causes include:

Kidney problems: Conditions such as chronic kidney disease, kidney artery narrowing (renal artery stenosis), or hormonal imbalances (such as primary aldosteronism or Cushing's syndrome) can lead to secondary hypertension. The kidneys play a vital role in regulating blood pressure by controlling the balance of salt and water in the body. When the kidneys are not functioning properly, blood pressure can rise.

Adrenal gland disorders: Conditions affecting the adrenal glands, such as excess production of hormones like aldosterone or cortisol, can contribute to high blood pressure. These hormones regulate salt and water balance in the body, and when their production is abnormal, blood pressure can increase.

Thyroid problems: An overactive thyroid gland (hyperthyroidism) or an underactive thyroid gland (hypothyroidism) can be associated with hypertension. Thyroid hormones influence the body's metabolism, including heart rate and blood vessel function. Imbalances in thyroid hormone levels can affect blood pressure regulation.

Certain medications: Certain medications, such as nonsteroidal anti-inflammatory drugs (NSAIDs), birth control pills, decongestants, and some antidepressants, can elevate blood pressure. It is important to discuss potential side effects with healthcare providers and monitor blood pressure regularly when taking these medications.

Other medical conditions: Sleep apnea, a sleep disorder characterized by interrupted breathing during sleep, is associated with hypertension. The repeated drops in oxygen levels during sleep can lead to increased blood pressure. Diabetes, certain tumors (pheochromocytoma), and certain congenital heart defects are among the other conditions that can cause secondary hypertension.

It's important to note that hypertension is often a silent condition, meaning it may not have noticeable symptoms. Regular blood pressure checks are essential for early detection and management. Lifestyle modifications, such as a healthy diet rich in fruits, vegetables, whole grains, and lean proteins, regular exercise, weight management, stress reduction techniques, and limiting alcohol and sodium intake, along with medication prescribed by a healthcare professional, are commonly recommended for managing high blood pressure. Early detection and management of high blood pressure can help prevent complications and improve overall health and well-being.

- Exploring the risk factors and genetic predispositions

Risk factors and genetic predispositions play a significant role in the development of high blood pressure. Understanding these factors can help individuals take proactive measures to prevent or manage hypertension. Here, we will explore the various risk factors and genetic influences associated with high blood pressure.

1. Age:
Advancing age is a significant risk factor for developing high blood pressure. As individuals get older, the blood vessels tend to become less flexible and more resistant to blood flow. This can lead to an increase in blood pressure. The risk of hypertension increases significantly after the age of 65.

2. Family History:
Having a family history of high blood pressure increases the risk of developing the condition. Genetic factors contribute to an individual's susceptibility to hypertension. If one or both parents have high blood pressure, the likelihood of developing the condition is higher. This suggests that there is a hereditary component to hypertension.

3. Ethnicity:

Certain ethnicities have a higher prevalence of high blood pressure. For example, African Americans tend to develop hypertension more frequently and at an earlier age compared to other racial or ethnic groups. Additionally, individuals of South Asian and Hispanic descent also have an increased risk of developing high blood pressure.

4. Gender:
Men are generally more prone to high blood pressure than premenopausal women. However, after menopause, the risk for women increases and becomes comparable to that of men. Hormonal changes during menopause, particularly a decrease in estrogen levels, may contribute to the development of hypertension in women.

5. Lifestyle Factors:
Unhealthy lifestyle choices can significantly increase the risk of developing high blood pressure. These factors include:

- Diet: A diet high in sodium (salt) and low in potassium can contribute to high blood pressure. Excessive sodium intake can cause the body to retain fluid, increasing blood volume and subsequently raising blood pressure. On the other hand, a diet rich in fruits, vegetables, whole grains, and low-fat dairy products, which are high in potassium, can help lower blood pressure.

- Physical Inactivity: Lack of regular physical activity can lead to weight gain and increase the risk of developing hypertension. Engaging in regular aerobic exercise, such as brisk walking or cycling, can help lower blood pressure and improve overall cardiovascular health.

- Obesity: Being overweight or obese puts extra strain on the heart and blood vessels, increasing the risk of hypertension. Excess body fat, particularly around the waistline, is associated with higher blood pressure levels.

- Tobacco Use: Smoking or using tobacco products can damage blood vessels, making them narrower and less flexible. This can lead to an increase in blood pressure. Additionally, exposure to secondhand smoke can also contribute to high blood pressure.

- Alcohol Consumption: Excessive alcohol consumption can raise blood pressure. It is recommended to limit alcohol intake to moderate levels, which is defined as up to one drink per day for women and up to two drinks per day for men.

6. Stress:
Chronic stress can contribute to the development of high blood pressure. When individuals are under stress, their body releases stress hormones that temporarily increase blood pressure. Prolonged or frequent stress can lead to sustained high blood pressure levels.

7. Genetic Predisposition:
Genetic factors contribute to an individual's susceptibility to high blood pressure. Several genes and gene variants have been identified as potential contributors to hypertension. These genes are involved in regulating blood vessel function, salt and water balance, and hormonal regulation. However, it is important to note that genetic predisposition is not a guarantee of developing hypertension. Environmental factors and lifestyle choices also play a significant role in the development of the condition.

In conclusion, high blood pressure is influenced by a combination of risk factors and genetic predispositions. Age, family history, ethnicity, gender, unhealthy lifestyle choices, stress, and genetic factors all contribute to the development of hypertension. Understanding these factors can help individuals make informed decisions regarding their lifestyle, adopt preventive measures, and seek appropriate medical care to manage high blood pressure effectively. It is important to consult with healthcare professionals for personalized advice and regular blood pressure monitoring to maintain optimal cardiovascular health.

- Discussing the connection between hypertension and other health conditions

Hypertension, or high blood pressure, is closely linked to several other health conditions. The relationship between hypertension and these conditions is often bidirectional, meaning that one condition can contribute to the development or worsening of the other. Understanding these connections is crucial for effective management and prevention strategies. In this discussion, we will explore the connection between hypertension and other health conditions.

1. Cardiovascular Diseases:
Hypertension is a significant risk factor for various cardiovascular diseases, including coronary artery disease, heart attack (myocardial infarction), heart failure, and stroke. When blood pressure is consistently high, it can damage the walls of the arteries, leading to the formation of plaques and narrowing of the blood vessels. This can restrict blood flow to the heart and other organs, increasing the risk of heart disease and stroke. Conversely, individuals with existing cardiovascular conditions are more likely to develop hypertension due to the strain on the heart and blood vessels.

2. Kidney Disease:
The kidneys play a vital role in regulating blood pressure by maintaining the balance of salt and water in the body. Hypertension can cause damage to the blood vessels in the kidneys, leading to reduced kidney function. Conversely, chronic kidney disease can disrupt the body's ability to regulate blood pressure, causing hypertension. The combination of hypertension and kidney disease can worsen the progression of both conditions, leading to a vicious cycle.

3. Diabetes:
Hypertension and diabetes often coexist and share similar risk factors, such as obesity and an unhealthy lifestyle. People with diabetes are more likely to develop hypertension due to insulin resistance and other metabolic abnormalities. Hypertension, in turn, increases the risk of complications in individuals with diabetes, including heart disease, kidney disease, and diabetic retinopathy (damage to the blood vessels in the retina).

4. Metabolic Syndrome:

Metabolic syndrome is a cluster of conditions that includes hypertension, high blood sugar levels, abnormal cholesterol levels, and excess abdominal fat. These conditions often occur together and increase the risk of cardiovascular disease, stroke, and type 2 diabetes. The exact relationship between hypertension and metabolic syndrome is complex, with shared underlying mechanisms such as insulin resistance and chronic inflammation.

5. Sleep Apnea:
Sleep apnea is a sleep disorder characterized by interrupted breathing during sleep. Individuals with sleep apnea are at an increased risk of developing hypertension. The repeated drops in oxygen levels during sleep can lead to increased blood pressure. Hypertension, on the other hand, can worsen sleep apnea symptoms and increase the risk of cardiovascular complications.

6. Obesity:
Obesity is closely associated with hypertension. Excess body weight puts additional strain on the heart and blood vessels, leading to increased blood pressure. Adipose tissue, particularly abdominal fat, produces hormones and inflammatory substances that can interfere with blood pressure regulation. Weight loss and lifestyle modifications, including a healthy diet and regular physical activity, are essential for managing both obesity and hypertension.

7. Mental Health Disorders:
There is a bidirectional relationship between mental health disorders, such as anxiety and depression, and hypertension. Chronic stress, which is often associated with mental health conditions, can contribute to the development of hypertension. Conversely, the diagnosis of hypertension and the need for ongoing management can lead to increased stress and impact mental well-being. It is important to address both mental health and hypertension simultaneously for optimal overall health.

8. Osteoporosis:
While the connection between hypertension and osteoporosis is not fully understood, some studies suggest that there may be a link. Hypertension medications, particularly long-term use of thiazide

diuretics, may increase the risk of developing osteoporosis. Additionally, both conditions share common risk factors, such as age and unhealthy lifestyle choices. Further research is needed to fully understand the relationship between hypertension and osteoporosis.

In conclusion, hypertension is closely connected to several other health conditions, including cardiovascular diseases, kidney disease, diabetes, metabolic syndrome, sleep apnea, obesity, mental health disorders, and potentially osteoporosis. Understanding these connections is crucial for comprehensive management and prevention strategies. Lifestyle modifications, such as a healthy diet, regular physical activity, stress reduction techniques, weight management, and medication prescribed by healthcare professionals, are commonly recommended for managing hypertension and its associated conditions. It is important to consult with healthcare professionals for personalized advice and regular monitoring to maintain optimal health and well-being.

Chapter 2: The Silent Killer: Unveiling the Myths and Misconceptions

- Debunking common misconceptions about high blood pressure

High blood pressure, also known as hypertension, is a common medical condition that affects millions of people worldwide. It is characterized by persistently elevated blood pressure in the arteries, which can lead to serious health complications if left untreated. However, there are several misconceptions and misunderstandings about high blood pressure that can hinder proper management and prevention. In this discussion, we will debunk some of the most common misconceptions about high blood pressure.

Misconception 1: High blood pressure is only a concern for older individuals.
Fact: While it is true that the risk of developing high blood pressure increases with age, it can affect individuals of all age groups. High

blood pressure can occur in children, adolescents, and young adults due to various factors such as genetics, unhealthy lifestyle choices, and underlying medical conditions. It is important for individuals of all ages to monitor their blood pressure regularly and take necessary steps to maintain optimal cardiovascular health.

Misconception 2: High blood pressure is always accompanied by noticeable symptoms.
Fact: High blood pressure is often referred to as the "silent killer" because it usually does not cause noticeable symptoms until it reaches severe levels. Many people with high blood pressure are unaware of their condition until it is detected during routine medical check-ups or when complications arise. Regular blood pressure monitoring is crucial, especially for individuals with risk factors such as obesity, family history, or certain medical conditions.

Misconception 3: High blood pressure is caused only by stress.
Fact: While stress can temporarily elevate blood pressure, it is not the sole cause of hypertension. High blood pressure is a complex condition influenced by various factors, including genetics, age, family history, unhealthy lifestyle choices, underlying medical conditions, and certain medications. Stress management is undoubtedly important for overall well-being, but it is not the sole determinant of blood pressure levels.

Misconception 4: Only people with a family history of high blood pressure are at risk.
Fact: While having a family history of high blood pressure does increase the risk, it is not the sole determining factor. Unhealthy lifestyle choices, such as a poor diet, lack of physical activity, excessive alcohol consumption, and tobacco use, can significantly contribute to the development of high blood pressure. Additionally, factors like age, ethnicity, and certain medical conditions can also increase the risk of hypertension.

Misconception 5: Hypertension can be cured and permanently eliminated.
Fact: Unfortunately, high blood pressure cannot be cured. However, it can be effectively managed and controlled through lifestyle

modifications and, if necessary, medication. Lifestyle changes, such as adopting a healthy diet, engaging in regular physical activity, managing stress, limiting alcohol consumption, and avoiding tobacco use, can help lower and maintain blood pressure within a healthy range. It is important to understand that hypertension requires ongoing management and adherence to a healthy lifestyle.

Misconception 6: People with high blood pressure should avoid exercise.
Fact: Regular exercise is actually beneficial for individuals with high blood pressure. Engaging in aerobic exercises, such as brisk walking, swimming, or cycling, can help lower blood pressure, improve cardiovascular health, and manage weight. However, it is important to consult with a healthcare professional before starting any exercise program, especially if blood pressure levels are significantly elevated or if there are other underlying health conditions.

Misconception 7: Taking hypertension medication means I no longer need to make lifestyle changes.
Fact: Medication prescribed for high blood pressure is often an essential component of treatment, but it does not negate the need for lifestyle modifications. Lifestyle changes, such as adopting a healthy diet, reducing sodium intake, managing stress, engaging in regular physical activity, and maintaining a healthy weight, are crucial for long-term blood pressure control. Medication should be taken as prescribed by a healthcare professional, and any adjustments should be made in consultation with them.

Misconception 8: Individuals with high blood pressure must completely avoid sodium.
Fact: While reducing sodium intake is generally recommended for individuals with high blood pressure, it is not necessary to completely eliminate sodium from the diet. Sodium is an essential nutrient that plays a role in various bodily functions. The key is to consume sodium in moderation and be mindful of hidden sources of sodium in processed foods and restaurant meals. A balanced diet that includes fresh fruits, vegetables, whole grains, lean proteins, and low-fat dairy products can help maintain a healthy blood pressure.

Misconception 9: Natural supplements can effectively lower blood pressure.
Fact: While some natural supplements and herbal remedies may claim to lower blood pressure, their effectiveness and safety are not well-established. It is important to consult with a healthcare professional before taking any supplements, as they may interact with medications or have adverse effects. Lifestyle modifications and prescribed medication, if necessary, are the primary approaches for managing high blood pressure.

- Exploring the hidden dangers and long-term effects

Regular blood pressure monitoring is essential, even if blood pressure is under control. While high blood pressure itself can have immediate health consequences, such as an increased risk of heart attack, stroke, and kidney disease, there are also hidden dangers and long-term effects that can occur if hypertension is left unmanaged.

1. Organ Damage: Elevated blood pressure puts strain on the blood vessels throughout the body, including those in the heart, brain, kidneys, and eyes. Over time, this can lead to damage to these organs, increasing the risk of heart disease, heart failure, stroke, kidney disease, and vision problems.

2. Cardiovascular Disease: High blood pressure is a major risk factor for developing cardiovascular diseases, such as coronary artery disease, heart attack, and heart failure. The constant pressure on the arteries can cause them to become stiff and narrow, reducing blood flow to the heart and increasing the workload on the heart.

3. Kidney Disease: The kidneys play a crucial role in filtering waste products from the blood. When blood pressure is consistently high, it can damage the blood vessels in the kidneys and impair their ability to function properly. This can lead to chronic kidney disease or even kidney failure.

4. Stroke: High blood pressure is the leading cause of strokes. Uncontrolled hypertension can cause blood vessels in the brain to weaken, rupture, or become blocked, depriving the brain of oxygen

and nutrients. This can result in a stroke, which can have serious and long-lasting effects on a person's health and quality of life.

5. Cognitive Decline: Research suggests that high blood pressure may contribute to cognitive decline and an increased risk of dementia, including Alzheimer's disease. The exact mechanisms are not fully understood, but it is believed that hypertension can damage blood vessels in the brain and impair cognitive function over time.

6. Eye Problems: High blood pressure can cause damage to the blood vessels in the eyes, leading to vision problems or even vision loss. Hypertensive retinopathy is a condition characterized by changes in the blood vessels in the retina, which can result in blurred vision, visual disturbances, or complete loss of vision.

7. Sexual Dysfunction: Uncontrolled high blood pressure can affect sexual function in both men and women. In men, it can contribute to erectile dysfunction by affecting blood flow to the penis. In women, it can lead to decreased sexual desire and difficulty achieving orgasm.

8. Sleep Apnea: High blood pressure and sleep apnea often go hand in hand. Sleep apnea is a condition characterized by interrupted breathing during sleep, which can lead to episodes of low oxygen levels and increased blood pressure. The combination of high blood pressure and sleep apnea can significantly increase the risk of cardiovascular events, such as heart attack and stroke.

9. Mental Health Issues: Chronic high blood pressure can also have an impact on mental health. Studies have shown a link between hypertension and an increased risk of depression, anxiety, and cognitive impairment. Managing blood pressure can not only improve physical health but also contribute to overall mental well-being.

10. Reduced Life Expectancy: If left uncontrolled, high blood pressure can significantly reduce life expectancy. The increased risk of cardiovascular disease, stroke, kidney disease, and other complications associated with hypertension can shorten a person's

lifespan. However, by managing blood pressure through lifestyle changes and appropriate medication, individuals can reduce their risk and improve their overall health and longevity.

It is important to debunk the misconception that high blood pressure is a benign condition or something that can be ignored. The hidden dangers and long-term effects of uncontrolled hypertension emphasize the importance of regular blood pressure monitoring, lifestyle modifications, and adherence to prescribed medication to effectively manage and prevent complications. By taking proactive steps to control blood pressure, individuals can significantly reduce their risk of these hidden dangers and improve their long-term health outcomes.

- Highlighting the importance of early detection and regular monitoring

Early detection and regular monitoring of blood pressure are crucial for managing and preventing the complications associated with high blood pressure. Here are the key reasons why early detection and regular monitoring are so important:

1. Identifying the Problem: High blood pressure is often referred to as the "silent killer" because it typically does not cause noticeable symptoms until it reaches severe levels. Without regular monitoring, individuals may be unaware that they have high blood pressure and may not seek the necessary medical attention. Early detection through regular blood pressure checks allows for timely intervention and management.

2. Preventing Complications: High blood pressure puts strain on the arteries and organs, increasing the risk of serious complications such as heart disease, stroke, kidney disease, and vision problems. Regular monitoring allows healthcare professionals to assess blood pressure levels and make recommendations for lifestyle changes and medication if necessary. By keeping blood pressure under control, the risk of complications can be significantly reduced.

3. Tailoring Treatment: Blood pressure can vary throughout the day, and regular monitoring helps determine the average blood pressure levels over time. This information is essential for healthcare professionals to tailor the treatment plan to an individual's specific needs. It allows for adjustments in medication dosage, lifestyle modifications, and other interventions to ensure optimal blood pressure control.

4. Tracking Progress: Regular monitoring provides a way to track progress and evaluate the effectiveness of lifestyle changes and medication in managing blood pressure. It allows individuals and healthcare professionals to see if the current treatment plan is working or if adjustments need to be made. It also helps motivate individuals by showing the positive impact of their efforts on their blood pressure levels.

5. Awareness and Education: Regular monitoring raises awareness about blood pressure and its importance in maintaining overall health. It provides an opportunity for individuals to learn about their own blood pressure patterns, risk factors, and the lifestyle modifications that can help manage hypertension. This knowledge empowers individuals to take control of their health and make informed decisions.

6. Early Intervention: Regular monitoring enables early intervention in case blood pressure levels start to rise. By detecting changes in blood pressure at an early stage, individuals can take immediate action to lower their blood pressure through lifestyle changes, stress management, and other strategies. Early intervention is key to preventing the progression of high blood pressure and reducing the risk of complications.

7. Encouraging Accountability: Regular monitoring creates a sense of accountability for individuals in managing their blood pressure. It serves as a reminder to prioritize their health and take the necessary steps to control their blood pressure. By consistently monitoring blood pressure, individuals are more likely to adhere to lifestyle modifications and medication, leading to better long-term outcomes.

In conclusion, early detection and regular monitoring of blood pressure are essential for managing and preventing the complications associated with high blood pressure. By staying proactive and aware of blood pressure levels, individuals can take control of their health, make necessary lifestyle changes, and work closely with healthcare professionals to maintain optimal blood pressure control. Regular monitoring is a vital tool in promoting long-term cardiovascular health and overall well-being.

Chapter 3: Lifestyle Factors and Hypertension

- Exploring the role of diet and nutrition in managing blood pressure

Diet and nutrition play a significant role in managing blood pressure. Making healthy food choices and adopting a balanced diet can help lower blood pressure levels and reduce the risk of hypertension-related complications. Here are some key dietary factors to consider:

1. Sodium Intake: High sodium intake is strongly associated with elevated blood pressure. Reducing the consumption of processed and packaged foods, which are typically high in sodium, is crucial. Instead, opt for fresh, whole foods and use herbs, spices, and other flavorings to enhance the taste of meals. It is recommended to limit sodium intake to less than 2,300 milligrams per day, or even lower for individuals with hypertension or other health conditions.

2. Potassium-Rich Foods: Potassium helps counteract the negative effects of sodium on blood pressure. Including potassium-rich foods in the diet can help lower blood pressure levels. Good sources of potassium include fruits (such as bananas, oranges, and avocados), vegetables (such as leafy greens, potatoes, and tomatoes), and legumes (such as beans and lentils).

3. Magnesium-Rich Foods: Magnesium plays a role in regulating blood pressure and relaxing blood vessels. Consuming foods high in

magnesium, such as leafy greens, nuts, seeds, whole grains, and legumes, can be beneficial for blood pressure management.

4. Calcium-Rich Foods: Calcium also plays a role in blood pressure regulation. Including low-fat dairy products (such as milk, yogurt, and cheese), fortified plant-based milk alternatives, leafy greens, and tofu in the diet can contribute to adequate calcium intake.

5. Healthy Fats: Choosing healthy fats over saturated and trans fats can have a positive impact on blood pressure. Incorporate sources of unsaturated fats, such as olive oil, avocados, nuts, and seeds, while limiting saturated and trans fats found in fried foods, fatty meats, and processed snacks.

6. Whole Grains: Whole grains, such as brown rice, quinoa, whole wheat bread, and oats, are rich in fiber and can help lower blood pressure. Aim to make at least half of the grains consumed whole grains.

7. Limit Alcohol Consumption: Drinking excessive amounts of alcohol can raise blood pressure. If alcohol is consumed, it is recommended to do so in moderation, which means up to one drink per day for women and up to two drinks per day for men.

8. Reduce Added Sugars: High intake of added sugars can contribute to weight gain and increased blood pressure. Minimize the consumption of sugary drinks, desserts, and processed snacks. Instead, choose natural sources of sweetness like fruits.

9. DASH Diet: The Dietary Approaches to Stop Hypertension (DASH) diet is an eating plan specifically designed to lower blood pressure. It emphasizes fruits, vegetables, whole grains, lean proteins, and low-fat dairy products. The DASH diet also encourages reducing sodium intake and limiting foods high in saturated fats and added sugars.

10. Portion Control: Managing portion sizes can help control calorie intake and maintain a healthy weight, which is important for blood pressure management. Use smaller plates and bowls, practice mindful eating, and listen to your body's hunger and fullness cues.

It is important to note that dietary changes alone may not be sufficient to manage high blood pressure, especially in cases of severe hypertension. It is recommended to work closely with a healthcare professional or registered dietitian to develop a personalized dietary plan based on individual needs and medical conditions. Regular blood pressure monitoring and medication adherence, if prescribed, are also essential components of overall blood pressure management.

- Discussing the impact of sedentary lifestyle and lack of physical activity

A sedentary lifestyle and lack of physical activity can have a significant impact on overall health, including an increased risk of developing high blood pressure. Here are some key points to consider regarding the impact of a sedentary lifestyle:

1. Increased Blood Pressure: Physical activity helps keep blood vessels healthy, improves blood flow, and lowers blood pressure. When individuals lead sedentary lives and engage in minimal physical activity, their blood pressure levels tend to be higher. Regular exercise can help lower blood pressure and reduce the risk of hypertension.

2. Weight Gain and Obesity: A sedentary lifestyle often leads to weight gain and obesity, which are major risk factors for high blood pressure. Lack of physical activity can contribute to an imbalance between calorie intake and expenditure, resulting in excess weight. Obesity puts additional strain on the heart and blood vessels, leading to higher blood pressure levels.

3. Poor Cardiovascular Health: Regular physical activity is crucial for maintaining cardiovascular health. When individuals are sedentary, the heart and blood vessels become less efficient at pumping blood, leading to a decrease in overall cardiovascular fitness. This can contribute to higher blood pressure and an increased risk of heart disease, stroke, and other cardiovascular complications.

4. Insulin Resistance and Metabolic Syndrome: Sedentary behavior is associated with an increased risk of insulin resistance and metabolic syndrome, both of which can contribute to the development of high blood pressure. Insulin resistance impairs the body's ability to effectively use insulin, leading to elevated blood sugar levels and an increased risk of hypertension. Metabolic syndrome is a cluster of conditions, including high blood pressure, high blood sugar, high cholesterol, and excess abdominal fat, which significantly increase the risk of cardiovascular disease.

5. Reduced Stress Management: Physical activity is a natural stress reliever. It helps reduce the levels of stress hormones, such as cortisol, and promotes the release of endorphins, which elevate mood and improve overall well-being. In contrast, a sedentary lifestyle can contribute to chronic stress, which can raise blood pressure levels over time.

6. Muscle Weakness and Loss: Lack of physical activity can lead to muscle weakness and loss of muscle mass. Muscles play an important role in supporting the joints and maintaining good posture. When muscles are weak or inactive, it can lead to poor posture and an increased risk of musculoskeletal problems, such as back pain or joint issues. This can further discourage individuals from engaging in physical activity, perpetuating a sedentary lifestyle.

7. Impact on Mental Health: Sedentary behavior has been linked to an increased risk of mental health conditions, such as depression and anxiety. These conditions can further contribute to a sedentary lifestyle and make it more challenging to engage in physical activity. Regular exercise, on the other hand, has been shown to improve mood, reduce symptoms of depression and anxiety, and enhance overall mental well-being.

To combat the negative effects of a sedentary lifestyle and lack of physical activity, it is important to incorporate regular exercise into daily routines. The American Heart Association recommends at least 150 minutes of moderate-intensity aerobic activity or 75 minutes of vigorous-intensity aerobic activity per week, along with muscle-strengthening activities at least two days per week. Even small changes, such as taking short walks during breaks, using stairs instead of elevators, or incorporating physical activity into leisure time, can make a significant difference. It is important to consult with a healthcare professional before starting any exercise program, especially if there are underlying health conditions or concerns.

- Providing strategies for stress management and its effect on blood pressure

Stress can have a significant impact on blood pressure levels. When individuals are stressed, their bodies release hormones that temporarily increase blood pressure. Prolonged or chronic stress can contribute to long-term high blood pressure and increase the risk of heart disease and other health problems. Here are some strategies for stress management and its effect on blood pressure:

1. Regular Exercise: Engaging in regular physical activity is a powerful stress-reliever. Exercise helps release endorphins, which are natural mood boosters. It also improves cardiovascular health, lowers blood pressure, and reduces the risk of chronic conditions. Aim for at least 150 minutes of moderate-intensity aerobic activity or 75 minutes of vigorous-intensity aerobic activity per week, along with muscle-strengthening activities.

2. Deep Breathing and Relaxation Techniques: Deep breathing exercises, such as diaphragmatic breathing or belly breathing, can activate the body's relaxation response, promoting a sense of calm and reducing stress. Other relaxation techniques, such as progressive muscle relaxation, guided imagery, or meditation, can also help manage stress and lower blood pressure. Find a technique that resonates with you and incorporate it into your daily routine.

3. Prioritize Sleep: Adequate sleep is essential for managing stress and maintaining overall health. Poor sleep quality or lack of sleep can contribute to increased stress levels and elevated blood pressure. Aim for 7-9 hours of quality sleep each night and establish a relaxing bedtime routine to promote better sleep.

4. Maintain a Healthy Diet: A balanced diet plays a crucial role in managing stress and blood pressure. Include plenty of fruits, vegetables, whole grains, lean proteins, and healthy fats in your meals. Avoid or limit the consumption of processed foods, sugary snacks, and excessive caffeine, which can exacerbate stress and affect blood pressure. Stay hydrated by drinking enough water throughout the day.

5. Practice Time Management: Poor time management can lead to increased stress levels. Prioritize tasks, set realistic goals, and break larger tasks into smaller, manageable steps. Learn to delegate when possible and avoid overcommitting yourself. Creating a structured schedule can help reduce stress and increase productivity.

6. Seek Social Support: Connecting with loved ones and building a support network is important for managing stress. Share your feelings and concerns with trusted friends or family members. Engage in activities that bring you joy and foster positive relationships. Join support groups or seek professional counseling if needed.

7. Engage in Stress-Relieving Activities: Find activities that help you relax and unwind. This can include hobbies like reading, listening to music, gardening, practicing yoga or tai chi, taking a warm bath, or spending time in nature. Engaging in activities you enjoy can help reduce stress levels and promote a sense of well-being.

8. Practice Mindfulness: Mindfulness involves paying attention to the present moment without judgment. It can help reduce stress and improve overall well-being. Incorporate mindfulness into your daily routine by practicing mindful eating, taking mindful walks, or using mindfulness apps or guided meditation.

9. Limit Exposure to Stressors: Identify and limit exposure to stressors that can be avoided. This may involve setting boundaries, managing your workload, or avoiding situations or people that trigger stress. Creating a peaceful and supportive environment can help reduce stress levels.

10. Seek Professional Help: If stress becomes overwhelming or interferes with daily functioning, it is important to seek help from a healthcare professional or therapist. They can provide guidance and support in managing stress and its impact on blood pressure.

Remember, stress management is a personal journey, and different strategies work for different individuals. It's essential to find what works best for you and make stress management a priority in your daily life.

Chapter 4: Unveiling the Hidden Culprits: Environmental and Occupational Factors

- Examining the impact of environmental factors on blood pressure

Environmental factors can have a significant impact on blood pressure levels. Here are some key environmental factors and their effects on blood pressure:

1. Air Pollution: Exposure to air pollution, particularly fine particulate matter (PM2.5), has been associated with increased blood pressure and a higher risk of hypertension. Air pollutants can enter the bloodstream and cause inflammation, oxidative stress, and damage to blood vessels, leading to elevated blood pressure levels.

2. Noise Pollution: Chronic exposure to high levels of noise, such as traffic noise or loud workplaces, has been linked to increased blood pressure. Noise pollution activates the body's stress response, leading to the release of stress hormones that can temporarily raise blood pressure. Prolonged exposure to noise pollution can contribute to long-term hypertension.

3. Temperature: Extreme temperatures, both hot and cold, can affect blood pressure. In hot weather, the body tries to cool down by dilating blood vessels, which can temporarily lower blood pressure. However, prolonged exposure to high temperatures can lead to

dehydration and increased blood viscosity, potentially raising blood pressure. Cold temperatures can cause blood vessels to constrict, increasing blood pressure.

4. Sodium Intake: High sodium intake, often associated with a Western diet and processed foods, can contribute to elevated blood pressure. Excess sodium causes the body to retain water, increasing blood volume and putting additional strain on blood vessels. It is important to monitor and reduce sodium intake to maintain healthy blood pressure levels.

5. Physical Environment: The physical environment in which individuals live and work can impact blood pressure. Factors such as access to green spaces, availability of recreational facilities, walkability of neighborhoods, and proximity to sources of environmental stress (e.g., industrial areas, high-traffic roads) can influence physical activity levels and stress levels, thereby affecting blood pressure.

6. Socioeconomic Factors: Socioeconomic factors, such as income level, education, and social support, can indirectly influence blood pressure. Lower socioeconomic status is often associated with higher levels of stress, limited access to healthcare, unhealthy lifestyle behaviors, and exposure to environmental stressors, all of which can contribute to elevated blood pressure.

7. Workplace Factors: Work-related stress and job strain can contribute to increased blood pressure. High-demand, low-control jobs, long working hours, shift work, and a lack of social support in the workplace can all contribute to chronic stress and elevated blood pressure levels. Occupational health and safety measures are important in managing workplace-related impacts on blood pressure.

8. Social Environment: The social environment, including family dynamics, relationships, and social support, can play a role in blood pressure regulation. Positive social interactions and strong social support networks have been associated with lower blood pressure levels, while social isolation and lack of support can contribute to higher blood pressure.

9. Access to Healthcare: Limited access to healthcare services and preventive measures can hinder the early detection and management of high blood pressure. Individuals with limited access to healthcare may have delayed or inadequate blood pressure monitoring, diagnosis, and treatment, increasing the risk of uncontrolled hypertension.

It is important to note that while these environmental factors can influence blood pressure, they interact with individual characteristics and lifestyle factors. Adopting a healthy lifestyle, including regular exercise, a balanced diet, stress management techniques, and regular blood pressure monitoring, can help mitigate the impact of environmental factors on blood pressure. Additionally, public health efforts, such as reducing air pollution, promoting green spaces, and improving access to healthcare, can contribute to the prevention and management of hypertension at a population level.

- Exploring the connection between occupation and hypertension

Occupation and hypertension, also known as high blood pressure, have been found to be interconnected. Numerous studies have examined the association between occupation and the risk of developing hypertension. The nature and demands of different occupations can contribute to the development and progression of hypertension. This article will explore the connection between occupation and hypertension, highlighting the factors that influence this relationship.

Several occupational factors can contribute to the development of hypertension. One significant factor is job strain, which refers to a combination of high job demands and low job control. Individuals in high-stress occupations, such as healthcare, law enforcement, and customer service, often experience high job demands and limited control over their work. The chronic stress associated with these occupations can lead to elevated blood pressure levels over time.

Shift work is another occupational factor associated with an increased risk of hypertension. Workers who regularly rotate between day, evening, and night shifts disrupt their circadian rhythm, which can negatively impact blood pressure regulation. The irregular sleep patterns, altered meal times, and exposure to artificial light during the night can disrupt the body's natural physiological processes, potentially leading to hypertension.

Sedentary occupations, where individuals spend a significant amount of time sitting or have limited physical activity, have also been linked to a higher risk of hypertension. Jobs that involve prolonged periods of sitting, such as office work or driving, can contribute to weight gain, obesity, and metabolic disturbances, all of which are risk factors for hypertension.

Occupational exposure to noise has also been associated with hypertension. Individuals working in noisy environments, such as construction sites or manufacturing plants, are exposed to high levels of noise pollution, which can activate the body's stress response. The release of stress hormones can temporarily elevate blood pressure, and chronic exposure to noise pollution can lead to sustained hypertension.

Work-related psychosocial factors, such as job insecurity, long working hours, and lack of social support, have also been identified as contributors to hypertension. Job insecurity and long working hours can lead to chronic stress, which in turn can affect blood pressure regulation. Additionally, a lack of social support in the workplace can further exacerbate the impact of occupational stress on blood pressure.

Certain occupational groups have been found to have a higher prevalence of hypertension. For example, healthcare workers, including nurses and physicians, often experience high levels of occupational stress and long working hours, putting them at increased risk of hypertension. Similarly, individuals in high-demand professions, such as executives and managers, may face job strain and a higher risk of hypertension.

On the other hand, some occupations have been associated with a lower risk of hypertension. Jobs that involve physical activity, such as construction work, agriculture, or active transportation, have been found to have a protective effect against hypertension. Regular physical activity can help maintain a healthy weight, improve cardiovascular fitness, and lower blood pressure.

Addressing the connection between occupation and hypertension requires a multi-faceted approach. Employers can play a crucial role in promoting employee health and reducing the risk of hypertension. Implementing workplace wellness programs that encourage physical activity, stress management techniques, and healthy lifestyle choices can be beneficial. Providing flexibility in work schedules and promoting work-life balance can also help mitigate the stress associated with certain occupations.

Individuals can take proactive steps to reduce their risk of hypertension in the workplace. Engaging in regular physical activity during breaks, incorporating stress management techniques such as deep breathing or mindfulness, maintaining a healthy diet, and seeking social support can all contribute to better blood pressure control.

In conclusion, occupation and hypertension are interconnected, with various occupational factors influencing the risk of developing hypertension. Job strain, shift work, sedentary work, exposure to noise, and work-related psychosocial factors can all contribute to elevated blood pressure levels. It is important for individuals and employers to prioritize strategies that promote a healthy work environment, including physical activity, stress management, and social support, to reduce the risk of hypertension among workers. By addressing the occupational factors that contribute to hypertension, individuals can strive for better overall health and well-being in the workplace.

- Discussing the importance of a healthy work-life balance

Maintaining a healthy work-life balance is crucial for overall well-being and success in both personal and professional aspects of life. It involves effectively managing time and energy between work responsibilities and personal activities, such as family, hobbies, self-care, and social connections. Here are some key reasons why a healthy work-life balance is important:

1. Physical and Mental Health: A healthy work-life balance helps prevent burnout and reduces the risk of physical and mental health issues. Chronic stress from an imbalance between work and personal life can lead to exhaustion, anxiety, depression, and other health problems. Taking time for self-care, relaxation, and pursuing hobbies can promote better physical and mental well-being.

2. Improved Productivity and Performance: When individuals have time for rest, relaxation, and pursuing personal interests, they return to work feeling refreshed and energized. This rejuvenation enhances focus, motivation, and productivity levels, leading to better job performance and efficiency. Taking breaks and having time for personal activities also allows for creativity and problem-solving skills to flourish.

3. Enhanced Relationships: A healthy work-life balance allows individuals to invest time and effort into building and maintaining meaningful relationships with family, friends, and loved ones. Spending quality time with loved ones strengthens bonds and provides emotional support, which is essential for overall happiness and well-being. It also helps in creating a support system during challenging times.

4. Personal Growth and Development: Engaging in personal activities and pursuing interests outside of work is essential for personal growth and development. It allows individuals to explore new hobbies, learn new skills, and expand their knowledge and experiences. Taking time for personal growth fosters a sense of fulfillment, self-confidence, and a broader perspective on life.

5. Stress Reduction and Work Satisfaction: Balancing work and personal life helps reduce stress levels. Constantly being overwhelmed with work can lead to increased stress and job dissatisfaction. On the other hand, having time for personal activities and relaxation provides a sense of control, reduces stress, and increases overall job satisfaction.

6. Setting a Positive Example: Maintaining a healthy work-life balance sets a positive example for colleagues, friends, and family. It promotes the importance of self-care, personal boundaries, and prioritizing well-being. By practicing work-life balance, individuals can encourage others to adopt healthier lifestyles and create a more supportive and balanced work culture.

-Tips for Achieving a Healthy Work-Life Balance:

1. Prioritize and set boundaries: Identify priorities in both work and personal life and set boundaries to ensure that time and energy are allocated accordingly. Learn to say no to excessive work demands when necessary.

2. Establish a routine: Create a schedule that includes dedicated time for work, personal activities, and relaxation. Stick to this routine as much as possible to maintain balance and avoid excessive work hours.

3. Delegate and seek support: Learn to delegate tasks at work and ask for help when needed. This will prevent becoming overwhelmed and provide opportunities for others to contribute.

4. Unplug and disconnect: Take regular breaks from technology and work-related communication, especially during personal time. Disconnecting from work allows for relaxation and rejuvenation.

5. Practice self-care: Engage in activities that promote physical and mental well-being, such as exercise, meditation, hobbies, and spending time in nature. Prioritize self-care as an essential part of maintaining work-life balance.

6. Communicate and negotiate: Openly communicate with supervisors, colleagues, and family members about your need for work-life balance. Negotiate flexible work arrangements, if possible, that align with personal needs and priorities.

Remember, achieving a healthy work-life balance is an ongoing process that requires conscious effort and regular evaluation. It may require adjustments and adaptations as personal and professional circumstances change. By prioritizing work-life balance, individuals can lead more fulfilling lives, experience greater overall happiness, and achieve long-term success in all areas of life.

Chapter 5: The Power of Medication: Understanding Treatment Options

- Exploring different types of medications used to manage high blood pressure

There are several types of medications available to manage high blood pressure, also known as hypertension. These medications work in different ways to lower blood pressure and reduce the risk of complications associated with hypertension. It's important to note that the choice of medication depends on individual factors, including the severity of hypertension, overall health, and any other existing medical conditions. Here are some common types of medications used to manage high blood pressure:

1. Diuretics: Diuretics, also known as water pills, are often prescribed as the first line of treatment for hypertension. They help the body eliminate excess sodium and water, reducing the volume of blood and decreasing blood pressure. Diuretics can be thiazide diuretics, such as hydrochlorothiazide, or loop diuretics, such as furosemide.

2. Angiotensin-Converting Enzyme (ACE) Inhibitors: ACE inhibitors work by blocking the production of angiotensin II, a hormone that narrows blood vessels and causes blood pressure to rise. By blocking this hormone, ACE inhibitors help relax and widen blood vessels, reducing blood pressure. Examples of ACE inhibitors include lisinopril, enalapril, and ramipril.

3. Angiotensin II Receptor Blockers (ARBs): ARBs work by blocking the action of angiotensin II at specific receptor sites, preventing it from constricting blood vessels. This leads to relaxation and widening of blood vessels, lowering blood pressure. Common ARBs include losartan, valsartan, and irbesartan.

4. Calcium Channel Blockers (CCBs): Calcium channel blockers prevent calcium from entering the smooth muscle cells of blood vessels and the heart. This relaxes and widens the blood vessels, reducing blood pressure. CCBs can be further classified into two subtypes: dihydropyridine (e.g., amlodipine, nifedipine) and non-dihydropyridine (e.g., diltiazem, verapamil).

5. Beta-Blockers: Beta-blockers reduce blood pressure by blocking the effects of adrenaline (epinephrine) on the heart and blood vessels. This slows down the heart rate, reduces the force of contraction, and lowers blood pressure. Beta-blockers commonly prescribed for hypertension include metoprolol, atenolol, and propranolol.

6. Alpha-Blockers: Alpha-blockers work by blocking certain receptors in the sympathetic nervous system, which helps relax and widen blood vessels, thereby lowering blood pressure. They may also reduce the tone of smooth muscles in the bladder and prostate. Examples of alpha-blockers include doxazosin, prazosin, and terazosin.

7. Renin Inhibitors: Renin inhibitors, such as aliskiren, work by directly inhibiting renin, an enzyme involved in the production of angiotensin II. By blocking renin, these medications reduce the production of angiotensin II, leading to relaxation and widening of blood vessels, and lowering blood pressure.

8. Alpha-2 Agonists: Alpha-2 agonists, like clonidine and methyldopa, work by stimulating certain receptors in the brain, which reduces the signals that increase blood pressure. These medications are often used in combination with other antihypertensive drugs.

In some cases, a combination of medications from different classes may be prescribed to effectively manage hypertension. It's important to follow the prescribed treatment plan, take medications as directed, and regularly monitor blood pressure to ensure it remains within a healthy range. It's also essential to consult a healthcare professional for personalized advice and guidance on medication options for managing high blood pressure.

- Discussing the benefits, side effects, and precautions of each medication

Here's a discussion on the benefits, side effects, and precautions of each medication commonly used to manage high blood pressure:

1. Diuretics:
- Benefits: Diuretics help reduce blood volume and lower blood pressure by promoting the excretion of excess sodium and water. They are generally well-tolerated and effective, especially for people with fluid retention or mild to moderate hypertension.
- Side effects: Common side effects may include increased urination, dehydration, electrolyte imbalances (such as low potassium levels), and dizziness. However, these side effects can often be managed with proper monitoring and adjustments.
- Precautions: Diuretics may not be suitable for individuals with certain medical conditions, such as kidney problems or diabetes. Regular monitoring of electrolyte levels is necessary, especially for those taking diuretics long-term.

2. Angiotensin-Converting Enzyme (ACE) Inhibitors:
- Benefits: ACE inhibitors effectively lower blood pressure by relaxing and widening blood vessels. They may also have additional benefits for people with heart failure, diabetes, or kidney disease.
- Side effects: Common side effects include a persistent dry cough, dizziness, and an increased risk of high potassium levels. In rare cases, ACE inhibitors can cause allergic reactions or kidney problems.
- Precautions: ACE inhibitors are generally not recommended for pregnant women as they can cause harm to the fetus. Regular monitoring of kidney function and potassium levels is important while taking ACE inhibitors.

3. Angiotensin II Receptor Blockers (ARBs):

- Benefits: ARBs work similarly to ACE inhibitors by relaxing blood vessels. They are an alternative for those who cannot tolerate ACE inhibitors due to the persistent cough.
- Side effects: Side effects are generally mild and can include dizziness, headache, and an increased risk of high potassium levels. Allergic reactions and kidney problems are rare.
- Precautions: ARBs are also not recommended for pregnant women. Regular monitoring of kidney function and potassium levels is advised.

4. Calcium Channel Blockers (CCBs):
- Benefits: CCBs lower blood pressure by relaxing and widening blood vessels, and some types can also reduce heart rate. They are particularly effective for older adults and individuals with certain heart conditions.
- Side effects: Common side effects may include dizziness, headache, flushing, and swelling of the ankles. Constipation and low blood pressure can occur, but these side effects are usually mild.
- Precautions: CCBs may interact with certain medications, so it's important to inform healthcare providers about all other drugs being taken. Grapefruit juice can also interact with CCBs, affecting their effectiveness.

5. Beta-Blockers:
- Benefits: Beta-blockers slow down the heart rate and reduce the force of heart contractions, thereby lowering blood pressure. They are often prescribed for individuals with heart disease or certain heart rhythm disorders.
- Side effects: Common side effects include fatigue, dizziness, cold hands and feet, and a potential worsening of asthma symptoms. Beta-blockers may also mask signs of low blood sugar in people with diabetes.
- Precautions: Beta-blockers should be used with caution in individuals with asthma or certain lung conditions. Abruptly stopping beta-blockers can lead to a rebound effect, so they should be gradually tapered off under medical supervision.

6. Alpha-Blockers:

- Benefits: Alpha-blockers relax and widen blood vessels, helping to lower blood pressure. They may also be used to manage symptoms of an enlarged prostate.
- Side effects: Common side effects include dizziness, lightheadedness, and a potential risk of low blood pressure when standing up (orthostatic hypotension). Alpha-blockers can also cause nasal congestion, fatigue, and headaches.
- Precautions: Alpha-blockers can cause a sudden drop in blood pressure, especially with the first dose. It's important to take the medication as directed and be cautious when changing positions.

7. Renin Inhibitors:
- Benefits: Renin inhibitors lower blood pressure by reducing the production of angiotensin II. They are effective in combination with other antihypertensive medications.
- Side effects: Common side effects include diarrhea, cough, and an increased risk of high potassium levels. Renin inhibitors may also cause dizziness and fatigue.
- Precautions: Renin inhibitors should not be used during pregnancy. Regular monitoring of kidney function and potassium levels is necessary.

8. Alpha-2 Agonists:
- Benefits: Alpha-2 agonists reduce blood pressure by targeting receptors in the brain to decrease sympathetic nerve activity. They can be effective for individuals with resistant hypertension or certain medical conditions.
- Side effects: Common side effects include drowsiness, dry mouth, and dizziness. Alpha-2 agonists may also cause rebound hypertension if abruptly discontinued.
- Precautions: Alpha-2 agonists should be used with caution in individuals with a

- Addressing common concerns and misconceptions about medication

Here are some common concerns and misconceptions about medication for high blood pressure:

1. Myth: "I feel fine, so I don't need to take my medication."
- Fact: High blood pressure often has no noticeable symptoms,
which is why it is often called the "silent killer." Even if you feel
fine, it is crucial to take your medication as prescribed. High blood
pressure puts strain on your heart and blood vessels, increasing the
risk of heart disease, stroke, and other complications.

2. Concern: "I'm worried about the side effects of medication."
- Response: While medications can have side effects, not everyone
experiences them, and they are often mild and manageable. It's
important to discuss any concerns with your healthcare provider.
They can help choose the most appropriate medication with the
fewest potential side effects for your specific situation.

3. Myth: "Once I start taking medication, I'll have to take it for the
rest of my life."
- Fact: High blood pressure is a chronic condition, and in most cases,
medication is necessary to manage it effectively. Lifestyle changes,
such as a healthy diet and regular exercise, can help, but they may
not be enough on their own. It's important to follow your healthcare
provider's recommendations and continue taking medication as
prescribed to keep your blood pressure under control.

4. Concern: "I'm worried about becoming dependent on medication."
- Response: Medication for high blood pressure is not addictive. It is
used to manage a chronic condition and help reduce the risk of
complications. If you have concerns about long-term medication use,
discuss them with your healthcare provider. They can provide
information and reassurance about the importance and benefits of
ongoing treatment.

5. Myth: "Once I start taking medication, I can stop making lifestyle
changes."
- Fact: Medication is an important part of managing high blood
pressure, but it is not a substitute for healthy lifestyle choices.
Lifestyle changes, such as eating a balanced diet, maintaining a
healthy weight, exercising regularly, limiting alcohol intake, and
managing stress, are crucial for long-term blood pressure control.

Medication and lifestyle changes work together to optimize your overall health and well-being.

6. Concern: "I'm worried about the cost of medication."
- Response: The cost of medication can vary depending on factors such as insurance coverage and the specific medication prescribed. If cost is a concern, discuss it with your healthcare provider. They may be able to recommend more affordable options or help you explore assistance programs or generic alternatives.

7. Myth: "I can adjust my medication dosage on my own."
- Fact: It is essential to follow your healthcare provider's instructions regarding medication dosage. Modifying the dosage or stopping medication without medical guidance can be dangerous and may lead to uncontrolled high blood pressure. Always consult your healthcare provider before making any changes to your medication regimen.

Remember, managing high blood pressure requires a comprehensive approach that includes medication, lifestyle changes, and regular monitoring. Open communication with your healthcare provider is key to address any concerns or misconceptions you may have. They can provide personalized guidance and support to help you effectively manage your blood pressure and reduce the risk of complications.

Chapter 6: Alternative Approaches: Complementary and Natural Remedies

- Investigating alternative therapies and their impact on blood pressure

While medication is the most common and effective treatment for high blood pressure, there are alternative therapies that may help complement conventional treatments and potentially have a positive impact on blood pressure. It's important to note that alternative therapies should not replace prescribed medication but can be used as adjunct therapies under the guidance of a healthcare professional. Here are a few alternative therapies that have shown some promise in managing blood pressure:

1. Mindfulness-Based Stress Reduction (MBSR): MBSR involves practicing mindfulness meditation, yoga, and body awareness techniques to reduce stress. Chronic stress can contribute to high blood pressure, so managing stress levels may have a positive impact on blood pressure. Several studies have shown that MBSR can help lower blood pressure in individuals with hypertension.

2. Biofeedback: Biofeedback is a technique that uses electronic devices to provide real-time information about physiological processes in the body, such as heart rate and blood pressure. By learning to control these processes, individuals may be able to lower their blood pressure. Biofeedback has demonstrated some effectiveness in reducing blood pressure in certain individuals.

3. Acupuncture: Acupuncture involves the insertion of thin needles into specific points on the body. It is believed to help restore the balance of energy flow in the body. Some studies suggest that acupuncture may have a modest effect in reducing blood pressure, but more research is needed to confirm its effectiveness.

4. Dietary Approaches: Certain dietary approaches, such as the DASH (Dietary Approaches to Stop Hypertension) diet, have been shown to help lower blood pressure. The DASH diet emphasizes fruits, vegetables, whole grains, lean proteins, and low-fat dairy products while limiting sodium, saturated fats, and cholesterol. Additionally, incorporating foods rich in potassium, such as bananas, avocados, and leafy greens, may have a positive impact on blood pressure.

5. Physical Activity: Regular physical activity, such as aerobic exercises, can help lower blood pressure. Engaging in activities like brisk walking, swimming, cycling, or dancing for at least 150 minutes per week can have significant benefits for blood pressure management. Always consult with your healthcare provider before starting any exercise program.

6. Herbal Remedies: Some herbal remedies, such as garlic extract, hawthorn extract, and green tea, have been studied for their potential effects on blood pressure. However, it's important to note that herbal remedies can interact with medications and may not be suitable for everyone. Consult with a healthcare professional before using herbal remedies.

It's crucial to discuss alternative therapies with your healthcare provider to ensure they are safe and appropriate for your specific situation. They can provide guidance on incorporating these therapies into your overall treatment plan and monitor their impact on your blood pressure. Remember, alternative therapies should be used in conjunction with prescribed medication and lifestyle modifications for optimal blood pressure management.

- Discussing the role of herbal supplements, acupuncture, and mindfulness techniques

Let's discuss the role of herbal supplements, acupuncture, and mindfulness techniques in managing various health conditions, including their potential impact on blood pressure.

1. Herbal Supplements:
Herbal supplements are derived from plants and are often used as alternative or complementary therapies. Some popular herbal supplements used for managing blood pressure include garlic extract, hawthorn extract, and green tea. However, it's important to note that the effectiveness of herbal supplements for blood pressure management is still being studied, and the results are mixed.

- Garlic extract: Some research suggests that garlic extract may have a modest effect in lowering blood pressure, but more studies are needed to confirm its efficacy.

- Hawthorn extract: Hawthorn extract is believed to have cardiovascular benefits and may help lower blood pressure. However, more research is required to determine its effectiveness and safety.

- Green tea: Green tea contains compounds called catechins that have been associated with potential blood pressure-lowering effects. However, the evidence is limited and inconsistent, and it's important to consume green tea in moderation due to its caffeine content.

It's crucial to consult with a healthcare professional before starting any herbal supplements, as they can interact with medications and may not be suitable for everyone. They can provide personalized guidance and monitor their impact on your blood pressure.

2. Acupuncture:
Acupuncture is an ancient Chinese practice that involves the insertion of thin needles into specific points on the body. It is believed to help restore the balance of energy flow, known as Qi (chee). While the exact mechanisms are not fully understood, acupuncture may have a positive impact on blood pressure.

- Some studies suggest that acupuncture may help lower blood pressure by promoting relaxation, reducing stress levels, and improving blood circulation. However, more research is needed to establish its effectiveness and determine the optimal treatment protocols.

- It's important to note that acupuncture should be performed by a qualified and licensed practitioner. Consult with your healthcare provider to determine if acupuncture is a suitable adjunct therapy for your blood pressure management.

3. Mindfulness Techniques:
Mindfulness techniques, such as mindfulness-based stress reduction (MBSR) and meditation, aim to cultivate a present-moment awareness and non-judgmental acceptance of thoughts, feelings, and sensations. These techniques have been studied for their potential benefits in managing stress, which can indirectly impact blood pressure.

- Chronic stress is linked to elevated blood pressure, so reducing stress levels through mindfulness techniques may have a positive impact on blood pressure management.

- Research suggests that practicing mindfulness techniques can help lower blood pressure in individuals with hypertension, improve cardiovascular health, and enhance overall well-being. Mindfulness techniques can also complement other lifestyle modifications, such as exercise and healthy eating.

Incorporating mindfulness techniques into your daily routine can be beneficial, but it's important to note that they should not replace prescribed medication. Consult with your healthcare provider to determine the most suitable mindfulness techniques for your specific needs and to learn proper techniques and practices.

Remember, herbal supplements, acupuncture, and mindfulness techniques can be used as complementary therapies alongside conventional treatments for blood pressure management. It's crucial to discuss these options with your healthcare provider to ensure they are safe, appropriate, and compatible with your overall treatment plan.

- Highlighting the importance of consulting healthcare professionals before trying alternative approaches

It is crucial to emphasize the importance of consulting healthcare professionals before trying any alternative approaches, including herbal supplements, acupuncture, and mindfulness techniques. Here are some reasons why consulting with a healthcare professional is essential:

1. Individualized Assessment: Healthcare professionals have the knowledge and expertise to assess your specific health condition, medical history, and current medications. They can determine if a particular alternative approach is safe and suitable for your unique circumstances.

2. Potential Interactions: Alternative approaches, such as herbal supplements, may interact with prescription medications, potentially causing adverse effects or reducing the effectiveness of the prescribed treatment. Healthcare professionals can evaluate potential interactions and make appropriate recommendations.

3. Monitoring and Evaluation: Regular monitoring and evaluation of your health status, including blood pressure, is essential for effective management. Healthcare professionals can track the impact of alternative approaches on your blood pressure and make adjustments to your treatment plan as needed.

4. Evidence-Based Information: Healthcare professionals stay up-to-date with the latest research and evidence regarding alternative therapies. They can provide accurate and evidence-based information, helping you make informed decisions about incorporating alternative approaches into your treatment plan.

5. Safety Considerations: Some alternative therapies may have potential risks or contraindications for certain individuals or specific health conditions. Healthcare professionals can assess your medical history and provide guidance on the safety of alternative approaches.

6. Comprehensive Approach: Healthcare professionals take a comprehensive approach to your health. They consider various factors, such as lifestyle modifications, medication management, and alternative therapies, to develop a holistic treatment plan that addresses your overall well-being.

By consulting healthcare professionals, you can ensure that any alternative approaches you consider are integrated safely and effectively into your overall treatment plan. They can provide personalized guidance, monitor your progress, and make necessary adjustments to optimize your blood pressure management. Remember, healthcare professionals are your trusted partners in achieving and maintaining your health goals.

Chapter 7: Prevention is the Key: Lifestyle Changes for Long-term Health

- Providing actionable steps to prevent high blood pressure

Here are some actionable steps you can take to help prevent high blood pressure:

1. Maintain a Healthy Weight:
Maintaining a healthy weight is crucial for blood pressure management. If you are overweight or obese, losing even a small amount of weight can have a significant impact on reducing blood pressure. Aim for a body mass index (BMI) within the normal range (18.5-24.9) and consult with a healthcare professional for personalized weight management guidance.

2. Adopt a Balanced Diet:
Eating a balanced diet rich in fruits, vegetables, whole grains, lean proteins, and low-fat dairy products can help lower blood pressure. Reduce your intake of sodium (salt), saturated fats, and added sugars. Consider the Dietary Approaches to Stop Hypertension (DASH) eating plan, which emphasizes fruits, vegetables, whole grains, and low-fat dairy while limiting sodium.

3. Limit Sodium Intake:
Reducing your sodium intake can help lower blood pressure. Aim to consume less than 2,300 milligrams (mg) of sodium per day, or even less if you have hypertension or are at risk. Read food labels, choose low-sodium options, and limit processed and packaged foods, which are often high in sodium.

4. Engage in Regular Physical Activity:
Regular physical activity is essential for maintaining a healthy blood pressure level. Aim for at least 150 minutes of moderate-intensity aerobic exercise or 75 minutes of vigorous-intensity aerobic exercise per week. Additionally, incorporate strength training exercises at least twice a week. Consult with a healthcare professional before starting any exercise program.

5. Limit Alcohol Consumption:
Excessive alcohol consumption can raise blood pressure. If you choose to drink alcohol, do so in moderation. For men, limit to no more than two standard drinks per day, and for women, limit to one standard drink per day. One standard drink is defined as 14 grams of

pure alcohol, which is typically found in a 5-ounce glass of wine, 12-ounce beer, or 1.5-ounce distilled spirits.

6. Quit Smoking:
Smoking and exposure to secondhand smoke can raise blood pressure and damage blood vessels. Quitting smoking is one of the most important steps you can take to improve your overall health and lower your blood pressure. Seek support from healthcare professionals, support groups, or smoking cessation programs to help you quit.

7. Manage Stress:
Chronic stress can contribute to high blood pressure. Find healthy ways to manage stress, such as engaging in relaxation techniques (e.g., deep breathing, meditation, yoga), participating in enjoyable activities, getting enough sleep, and seeking support from friends, family, or a mental health professional.

8. Monitor Blood Pressure:
Regularly monitor your blood pressure to ensure it stays within a healthy range. Home blood pressure monitors are available for convenient monitoring. If you have concerns about your blood pressure readings, consult with a healthcare professional for further evaluation and guidance.

Remember, these steps are general recommendations, and it's important to consult with a healthcare professional for personalized advice based on your specific health condition and risk factors. By taking proactive measures and making positive lifestyle changes, you can help prevent high blood pressure and maintain overall cardiovascular health.

- Exploring the importance of regular exercise, healthy eating, and stress reduction

Regular exercise, healthy eating, and stress reduction are three key components of a healthy lifestyle, and their importance cannot be overstated. Let's explore each of these components in more detail:

1. Regular Exercise:

Regular physical activity offers numerous benefits for overall health and well-being, including blood pressure management. Here's why exercise is important:

- Blood Pressure Control: Engaging in regular exercise can help lower blood pressure and reduce the risk of developing hypertension. Exercise strengthens the heart, improves blood circulation, and helps maintain the flexibility and health of blood vessels.

- Weight Management: Exercise plays a crucial role in maintaining a healthy weight or achieving weight loss. It helps burn calories, build lean muscle mass, and increase metabolic rate, contributing to weight control and reducing the risk of obesity-related conditions, including high blood pressure.

- Stress Reduction: Exercise is a powerful stress reliever. Physical activity releases endorphins, which are natural mood-boosting chemicals in the brain. Regular exercise can help reduce stress, anxiety, and depression, promoting overall mental well-being.

- Cardiovascular Health: Exercise improves cardiovascular fitness, strengthens the heart muscle, and enhances the efficiency of the cardiovascular system. It can lower the risk of heart disease, stroke, and other cardiovascular conditions, including high blood pressure.

Aim for a combination of aerobic exercises (such as brisk walking, jogging, cycling, swimming) and strength training exercises (such as weightlifting, resistance training) for optimal benefits. Consult with a healthcare professional before starting any exercise program.

2. Healthy Eating:
A balanced and nutritious diet is essential for maintaining good health and managing blood pressure. Here's why healthy eating is important:

- Blood Pressure Management: A diet rich in fruits, vegetables, whole grains, lean proteins, and low-fat dairy products, and low in sodium, saturated fats, and added sugars can help lower blood pressure. The Dietary Approaches to Stop Hypertension (DASH) eating plan is specifically designed to promote heart health and lower blood pressure.

- Weight Control: Healthy eating, combined with portion control, can contribute to weight management or weight loss. Maintaining a healthy weight is crucial for blood pressure control, as excess weight can strain the cardiovascular system and increase the risk of hypertension.

- Nutrient Intake: A well-balanced diet provides essential nutrients, vitamins, and minerals necessary for overall health and the proper functioning of the body. These nutrients support cardiovascular health, immune function, and overall well-being.

- Disease Prevention: Healthy eating habits can help reduce the risk of various chronic diseases, including heart disease, diabetes, and certain types of cancer. By managing these underlying conditions, the risk of high blood pressure can also be minimized.

Aim for a diet that includes a variety of nutrient-dense foods, emphasizing fruits, vegetables, whole grains, lean proteins, and healthy fats. Limit sodium intake, choose foods low in saturated fats and added sugars, and drink plenty of water.

3. Stress Reduction:
Chronic stress can have a negative impact on blood pressure and overall health. Incorporating stress reduction techniques into your daily routine is vital. Here's why stress reduction is important:

- Blood Pressure Control: Prolonged stress can lead to increased blood pressure levels. Stress activates the body's "fight or flight" response, causing temporary increases in blood pressure. Chronic stress can disrupt this balance and contribute to sustained high blood pressure.

- Mental Well-being: High levels of stress can negatively affect mental health, leading to anxiety, depression, and other mental health disorders. Prioritizing stress reduction can improve overall mental well-being and quality of life.

- Healthy Coping Mechanisms: Engaging in stress reduction techniques, such as deep breathing exercises, meditation, yoga, mindfulness, and engaging in hobbies or activities you enjoy, can promote relaxation, improve mood, and reduce the harmful effects of stress on blood pressure.

- Lifestyle Habits: Stress management often involves adopting healthy lifestyle habits, such as regular exercise, adequate sleep, and maintaining social connections. These habits contribute to overall well-being and can help lower blood pressure.

Find stress reduction techniques that work for you and incorporate them into your daily routine. Experiment with different methods and seek support from healthcare professionals or mental health professionals if needed.

Remember, these lifestyle factors are interconnected, and adopting a holistic approach that includes regular exercise, healthy eating, and stress reduction is key to maintaining good health, managing blood pressure, and reducing the risk of chronic diseases. Consult with a healthcare professional for personalized guidance and recommendations based on your individual needs and health condition.

- Discussing the benefits of maintaining a healthy weight and managing other health conditions

Maintaining a healthy weight and managing other health conditions offer numerous benefits for overall well-being and can positively impact blood pressure. Let's explore the benefits of maintaining a healthy weight and managing other health conditions:

1. Maintaining a Healthy Weight:
Maintaining a healthy weight is important for several reasons, including blood pressure management. Here are some key benefits:

- Blood Pressure Control: Excess weight, especially around the waistline, can contribute to high blood pressure. Losing weight and maintaining a healthy weight can help lower blood pressure and reduce the risk of hypertension. It eases the strain on the heart and blood vessels, allowing them to function more efficiently.

- Reduced Risk of Chronic Diseases: Maintaining a healthy weight lowers the risk of various chronic diseases, including heart disease, type 2 diabetes, certain types of cancer, and respiratory conditions. These conditions can exacerbate high blood pressure or increase the risk of developing it.

- Improved Cardiovascular Health: Maintaining a healthy weight supports overall cardiovascular health. It reduces the risk of atherosclerosis (hardening of the arteries), improves blood circulation, and enhances the heart's ability to pump blood effectively.

- Enhanced Physical Functioning: Being at a healthy weight can improve physical functioning and mobility. It reduces the strain on joints, muscles, and bones, making it easier to engage in physical activities and maintain an active lifestyle.

- Increased Energy Levels: Maintaining a healthy weight can boost energy levels and overall vitality. When the body is at a healthy weight, it functions optimally, leading to increased energy and improved overall well-being.

2. Managing Other Health Conditions:
Managing other health conditions also plays a significant role in blood pressure management. Here are some benefits of effectively managing other health conditions:

- Diabetes Management: If you have diabetes, managing your blood sugar levels is crucial for blood pressure control. Consistently maintaining healthy blood sugar levels can help prevent complications, such as high blood pressure, and reduce the risk of cardiovascular diseases.

- Cholesterol Control: High cholesterol levels can contribute to the development of atherosclerosis and increase the risk of high blood pressure. Managing cholesterol levels through lifestyle changes and, if necessary, medication can help maintain optimal blood pressure levels.

- Kidney Disease Management: Chronic kidney disease can lead to high blood pressure. By effectively managing kidney disease through medication, dietary changes, and regular medical check-ups, the risk of high blood pressure can be minimized.

- Sleep Apnea Treatment: Sleep apnea, a condition characterized by interrupted breathing during sleep, can increase the risk of high blood pressure. Treatment options, such as continuous positive airway pressure (CPAP) therapy or lifestyle modifications, can help manage sleep apnea and improve blood pressure control.

- Stress Reduction: Chronic stress can contribute to high blood pressure. Adopting stress reduction techniques, such as exercise, relaxation techniques, and seeking support from healthcare professionals or mental health professionals, can help manage stress and positively impact blood pressure.

Effectively managing these health conditions through lifestyle modifications, medication, and regular medical care can have a positive impact on blood pressure control and overall health.

It's important to note that maintaining a healthy weight and managing other health conditions should be done under the guidance of healthcare professionals. They can provide personalized recommendations, create a comprehensive treatment plan, and monitor your progress to ensure optimal results.

By maintaining a healthy weight and effectively managing other health conditions, you can improve blood pressure control, reduce the risk of complications, and enhance overall well-being. Remember to consult with healthcare professionals for personalized advice based on your specific health condition and needs.

Conclusion:

Maintaining a healthy lifestyle and managing other health conditions are crucial for blood pressure management. Here are the key takeaways:

1. Regular Exercise:
- Engaging in regular exercise helps control blood pressure, manage weight, reduce stress, and improve cardiovascular health.
- Aim for a combination of aerobic exercises and strength training for optimal benefits.

2. Healthy Eating:
- Adopt a balanced and nutritious diet, such as the DASH eating plan, to manage blood pressure and weight.
- Emphasize fruits, vegetables, whole grains, lean proteins, and limit sodium, saturated fats, and added sugars.

3. Stress Reduction:
- Chronic stress can contribute to high blood pressure, so incorporate stress reduction techniques like deep breathing, meditation, and hobbies.
- Prioritize healthy coping mechanisms, lifestyle habits, and seek support if needed.

4. Maintaining a Healthy Weight:
- Maintaining a healthy weight helps control blood pressure, reduces the risk of chronic diseases, and improves cardiovascular health.
- It eases strain on the heart and enhances physical functioning and energy levels.

5. Managing Other Health Conditions:
- Effectively manage conditions like diabetes, high cholesterol, kidney disease, and sleep apnea to minimize the risk of high blood pressure.
- Seek medical guidance and follow treatment plans to optimize blood pressure control.

Overall, blood pressure management is essential for overall health and well-being. By adopting a holistic approach that includes regular exercise, healthy eating, stress reduction, maintaining a healthy weight, and managing other health conditions, you can reduce the risk of hypertension, improve cardiovascular health, and enhance your quality of life. Remember to consult with healthcare professionals for personalized guidance and support.

Taking control of your health and making positive lifestyle changes is within your reach. Here's why it's important and how you can start:

1. Empowerment and Ownership:
By taking control of your health, you become an active participant in your well-being. You have the power to make decisions and take actions that can positively impact your health and quality of life.

2. Prevention is Key:
Making positive lifestyle changes can help prevent the onset of chronic diseases, including high blood pressure. By adopting healthy habits, you reduce the risk of developing conditions that can affect your overall health.

3. Long-Term Benefits:
Positive lifestyle changes offer long-term benefits that go beyond just managing blood pressure. They contribute to improved cardiovascular health, increased energy levels, enhanced mental well-being, and reduced risk of other chronic diseases.

4. Start Small:
Begin by setting realistic and achievable goals. Start with small changes such as incorporating more fruits and vegetables into your diet, taking short walks, or practicing stress-reducing techniques. Gradually build on these habits to create a sustainable and healthy lifestyle.

5. Seek Support:
Don't hesitate to seek support from healthcare professionals, family, and friends. They can provide guidance, accountability, and encouragement along your health journey.

6. Stay Consistent:

Consistency is key when making positive lifestyle changes. Aim to make these changes a part of your daily routine rather than relying on temporary fixes. Remember, small steps taken consistently can lead to significant long-term improvements.

7. Celebrate Progress:
Acknowledge and celebrate your achievements, no matter how small they may seem. Recognize the positive changes you've made and the impact they have on your health and well-being.

By taking control of your health and making positive lifestyle changes, you can improve your blood pressure management, reduce the risk of chronic diseases, and enhance your overall quality of life. Start today, believe in yourself, and embrace the journey towards a healthier and happier you.

By providing accurate information, debunking myths, and offering practical solutions, "Unmasking Hypertension: The Truth About High Blood Pressure and Proven Solutions for Prevention" aims to empower readers to take control of their blood pressure and lead healthier lives.

Dear Reader's,

I wanted to take a moment to express my heartfelt gratitude for your engagement and interest in my book on Hypertension. Your dedication to expanding your knowledge in this area is truly commendable, and I hope that the information I provided has been helpful in your understanding of Hypertension

As an author, my ultimate goal is to provide valuable and insightful content that resonates with readers like yourself. Your support and feedback are incredibly important to me, as they help me improve my work and reach a wider audience.

I would be immensely grateful if you could take a few moments to leave an honest review of my book. Your review will not only help me understand what you found valuable or enjoyable about the book, but it will also guide other potential readers in making an informed decision. Your thoughts and experiences are valuable, and I believe they can make a real difference in the lives of others who are seeking guidance in this area.

I understand that leaving a review may take a little time and effort, but please know that your contribution will have a lasting impact. Your honest feedback will not only help me grow as an author but also assist others in making informed choices when it comes to Hypertension

Thank you once again for your support and for considering leaving a review. I truly appreciate your time and input.

Warmest regards,
M Livingston